T0169547

GOODBYE COMFORT FOOD

Advance Praise

"My clients with food issues are laughing and relating to this book in a way that brings them hope and supportive tools to use every day."

— **Wendi Carter**, LCSW, Counselor and Life Coach

"Robin's insights are like the combination of your best friend, confidant, expert and equal."

— **Dr. Deborah Walters**, author of *The Supreme Remedy*, www.deborahshealingarts.com

"This book has given me hope after years of struggle."

— **Linda**, client

GOODBYE COMFORT FOOD

How to FREE YOURSELF *From Overeating*

ROBIN RAE MORRIS

NEW YORK

LONDON • NASHVILLE • MELBOURNE • VANCOUVER

GOODBYE COMFORT FOOD
How to FREE YOURSELF *From Overeating*

Published in New York, New York, by Morgan James Publishing in partnership with Difference Press. Morgan James is a trademark of Morgan James, LLC. www.MorganJamesPublishing.com

ISBN 978-1-64279-280-5 paperback
ISBN 978-1-64279-281-2 eBook
Library of Congress Control Number: 2018911228

Cover Design by:
Rachel Lopez
www.r2cdesign.com

Interior Design by:
Bonnie Bushman
The Whole Caboodle Graphic Design

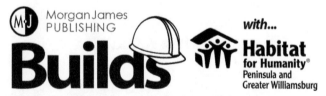

In an effort to support local communities, raise awareness and funds, Morgan James Publishing donates a percentage of all book sales for the life of each book to Habitat for Humanity Peninsula and Greater Williamsburg.

Get involved today! Visit
www.MorganJamesBuilds.com

For Nancy B. Jacobs,
who taught me about being shape-able.

Table of Contents

Favorite Comfort Foods and Why They are a Brilliant Choice

They don't call it comfort food for nothin'! Let's talk about what they are. C'mon, you know your mouth is already watering. Your mind is planning for when you'll eat them. You can feel it so close, so let's name names!

In no particular order, our cast of characters includes, but is not limited to:

- Fried chicken
- Teriyaki chicken
- Chicken alfredo
- Pasta with meatballs
- Pasta with tofu
- Pasta with parmesan
- Pizza with parmesan

- Brie, cheddar, or goat cheese on bread
- Sourdough bread, 14-grain bread, or cinnamon raisin English muffins
- Blueberry muffins, chocolate chip cookies, carrot cakes, and lemon pies
- Bacon and eggs. Bacon and everything.
- Fruit *

*Fruit. No. Just kidding. I once had a therapist tell me "If you have to eat for comfort, try eating fruit." I thought, *You just don't get it.*

And now I realize how much she didn't get it. Not only have I never met a single comfort food eater who wants to soothe with sliced fruit, the physiology isn't there.

Our go-to comfort foods of choice are brilliant. They are the foods that will dampen our physiology so that we literally feel less emotion and stress. Additionally, since most of our comfort food choices involve sugars and carbohydrates, our brains will begin to crave even more of them, which keeps us trapped in a comfort-food feedback loop that becomes progressively harder to break.

Then there's the marketing that surrounds us. A recent advertising poster outside of the local Starbucks featured a photo of a whipped cream topped caramel coffee drink below which was written, "Made to Crave." Like that's a good thing.

Well, maybe it is for Starbucks. Yet my point is that as if it weren't difficult enough to break a comfort food, emotional eating cycle, everywhere we look, we're encouraged to reward ourselves with foods that increase the very cravings we're trying to overcome. C'mon, "you deserve a break today." And you do, you deserve the opportunity to break away from foods and habits that momentarily sweeten your life, yet ultimately steal your soul, well-being, energy, and positive sense of self.

Speaking of giving yourself a break, before you go any further in this book, the first thing I'd like you to do is to congratulate yourself for choosing comfort food. It's a brilliant way to deal with the world: simple, effective, and efficient; a dependable problem with a dependable response and dependable outcome.

Something up? Something uncertain? Grab a two-foot submarine sandwich and down that puppy in one sitting. Go ahead. No one's judging. Ok. You might be judging yourself, but not in that moment, because in that moment, there is the experience of "yum, yum, yum, yum, yum, yum, yum" in every quickly inhaled bite.

Yes, we love comfort food. And we long for a way out of this mess. There is a way out of turning to food when life throws you a curveball, your boss expects overtime, your kids are a mess, and your life feels unmanageable.

There is also the possibility that, once a comfort food woman, the desire (whether quietly nudging you or urgently screaming at you) to turn to your favorite comfort food in times of trouble and turmoil will never completely go away.

What will change, I promise you and I know you don't and shouldn't believe me yet, is that no amount of comfort food will ever be worth your peace of mind, clarity of thoughts, and ease of taking fruitful action. (Which I guess is where the fruit actually comes in.)

Welcome to Heaven, Then Hell

2

Helen has had a hard day at the office. Despite a recent promotion that originally left her elated, she is now overwhelmed at no longer being part of the team, but instead giving her first performance reviews to people who used to be her co-workers and pals.

Her first performance review required putting a pal on a performance plan. It was a tense meeting. It ended in polite and politically correct statements addressed to one another. At the end of the meeting, Helen thought, "We used to share with one another. Now, we're speaking corporate speak—the kind of language we used to make fun of!" Helen felt the pang of lost connection.

Helen returned home, put on her PJs, skipped dinner, pulled out a pint of Ben and Jerry's Chocolate Therapy ice cream and a package of Walkers shortbread cookies shaped like adorable Scottish Terrier dogs, and cuddled up in a blanket on the couch. Netflix, and comfort food, take her away!

She simultaneously watched the newest installment of *This Is Us*, while the ice cream melted away her cares. The smooth, buttery cookies added just a bit of crunch. The creamy goodness and buttery crunch became one with the emotional catharsis of people living an intense TV life. Suddenly, Helen was in heaven.

She polished off another pint of ice cream, the entire package of cookies, and three more episodes before falling into bed in a kind of sluggish, tired coma.

Helen wakes the next morning with a surging sense of dread. She is going to have to go into work and do a second performance review. The terror about that has no immediate buffer, and since she overslept and is still feeling stuffed from the previous evening, there is no room, nor time, for food to comfort her now. She tries on three outfits before she finds one that semi-fits.

The things she thinks about herself as she looks in the mirror are demoralizing. She is anxious and grouchy and has a food-hangover. Suddenly, Helen is in hell.

Hell has been described as a fiery place where the bad get their comeuppance. Yet, people who use food as comfort know that h*** is everywhere, any time, you look at yourself in disgust and think, "I did it again."

Unknown to many is a second heaven. One that is arguably better than the first. This is a heaven that offers a ladder out of hell. Each rung of the ladder is a solidly defined step. Your task is to grab onto the ladder to advance to the next rung. Soon, yet not without effort, you will have arrived at your definition of living a life that is your heaven on earth.

This book will give you seven practices to help you climb out of hell. They are called practices because you can do them daily without having to quit your job, leave your family, join a monastery or a circus, or take any other extreme measures. For now, nothing has to change except for the faintest hope that there may be a way out of emotional eating. The way out is built on practice, which includes failure, bumps and starts, and truly delicious moments of success. The way out is built on practice, not perfection.

The Tyranny of Mind, Body, and Soul

I t all started in the summer between second and third grade. I spent six glorious weeks with my grandmother during which I learned the joys of freshly fried bread dough smeared with butter and dipped in sugar. I explored nightly the comfort that came from eating toasted tuna fish sandwiches before bedtime. These were made from thick slices of homemade white bread and eaten while watching *The Big Valley* television series. I'd eat the sandwich while nourishing my crush on Michael Landon. I returned home at the end of the summer. At my back to school visit with the pediatrician, he said that I had "gained too much weight for my height and age."

"I'm fat," I told my mother. "You're beautiful," she said.

It was a nice try on her part. Yet she wasn't fat, none of her friends were fat, and none of mine were either. My body—I—was different. The teasing from other kids and woeful, sobbing trips to the Sears Chubby Department to purchase clothing confirmed that this kind of different wasn't a good kind.

At thirteen, I decided enough was enough. Well, actually I decided enough was too much, and put myself on a 600 calorie a day diet. I remember being light headed if I stood up too fast and the silent pursed-lipped standoffs when my father would say, "Just eat." I remember trying to hide the fact that my fingernails started getting dents, then holes in them. Back to the pediatrician and lots of boiled liver for my efforts.

There must be a better way. I was stumped for a few years on this, yet eventually I cracked the code. Long before it was known and named, I came up with a spiffy way to eat everything I wanted—which was by then quite a lot due to many years of deprivation and diets—and not gain too much weight. My great insight into how to pull this off is known as bulimia, a form of overeating followed by purging. I'm not proud of this; yet at the time, it certainly seemed better than another starvation diet. And hey, no boiled liver.

After college and diets and disordered eating, I had come to a place where I wouldn't say I ate "normally," but I had figured out what worked for me. Part of learning to do that also helped me come up with a few shortcuts in other areas of my life. For instance, I learned that if a guy couldn't deal with the fact that

I would eat an apple in two to four sittings, it wasn't worth starting a relationship with him. But I digress.

I had graduated in psychology and had gotten my first career position as a counselor. I did not specialize in eating disorders. I felt I'd lived enough of that and found myself fascinated by the realms of psychosis and mania.

I remember visiting a client in the psych ward who had tried to strangle herself while manic. It was good to see her, and good to see her alive. Surviving the attempt had brought a new determination to deal with her mania and its life-crashing episodes. As I looked at her, I noticed that there were tiny red dots around her eyes.

"Your eyes?" I asked, after we had talked a bit.

Looking away from me, she said, "The strangulation attempt, it … it, um, cut off oxygen and burst blood vessels in my eyes."

Immediately I teared up. My heart ached for her and for myself too. I recalled a time, in my twenties, when I'd gone to the emergency department looking a lot like her. I had eaten so much that I vomited, hard, and repeatedly. I had those little red dots around my eyes.

It had never dawned on me that overeating was a way of strangling myself. Yet, looking at her, knowing the Universe had brought me a mirror of sorts, I knew this to be true down to my bones.

Overeating, or undereating, or whatever other compulsive forms my eating has taken, was a physical strangulation of my existence. It was right there in the eyes, the doorway to the soul.

It was a mental and emotional strangulation that cut me off from facing my thoughts, feelings, and beliefs when they were painful, uncomfortable, unsettling. It was a way of being in which I was convinced "I can't," so I stayed un-empowered and played small on the inside, in my internal world. It was a strangulation that cut me off from myself, and from anything one would call God or The Universe.

It was my first revelation of just how much distance there was between my deep internal longings for healthy eating, and what appeared to others on the outside. I could, at times, look like I played big, yet in actuality and in essence, I had learned to play, and stay, small. To stay within the tiny circumference of those small red dots.

From the opportunity to see clearly the self-imposed tyranny against my own body, came the beginnings of true freedom.

Freedom, and relief came in the form of working through eating issues with others. I attended workshops where we would laugh, cry, hug, and heal. I think it was the laughing that did it. It was sitting in a group of people, hearing one strange and slightly bizarre eating habit after another, all of which were simultaneously foreign and familiar, that led me to turn my counseling focus toward emotional eating.

After years of counseling clients and speaking to local organizations about how to refresh and refuel their lives, I had quite a tool kit. I realized it was time to open up that tool kit and create a program that would bring freedom to those suffering from emotional eating.

It began with a handful of clients. I showed up with seven practices and they showed up with willingness and a desire to get a result that had been eluding them. Together, we practiced and polished the program into the form you will find in this book, and the one that I teach both one on one and in groups. I found that learning a set of structured yet flexible daily practices helped clients create healthy eating habits, naturally lose weight, curb emotional eating, and gain positive energy.

In my first book, *Devour Obstacles for Dinner*, I lay out tools that can be used by anyone for a myriad of situations, such as resolving relationship issues, finding your passion, overcoming depression and anxiety symptoms, creating mindfulness practices, and achieving both long- and short-term goals.

This book you have in your hand is more specific. It is for you who suffer from out of balance eating. This book is the one in which we—you and I—journey together toward being as great at food as you are at all of the other amazing things you pull off in your life. We are talking about freedom from emotional eating.

This freedom is my wish for you, Brave One. This freedom, not despite your eating issues, yet actually because of and through them. This freedom, and the positive energy for your life and your path it will open. Are you ready to leave emotional eating behind and start playing big?

Kat, as all of Katrina's friends call her, is a woman who plays big. She's an awesome mom of two beautiful children, a wonderful and loving wife, a dedicated and successful manager. She's a fun and supportive friend, always there to host a party or lend a hand. By all external standards, she is playing big.

Until I ask her a question about self-care. Her normally animated face goes blank. I can hear the gears of her mental apparatus turning, trying to click-in to the question. Finally, she gives up answering it, and says this instead:

"Give me a role and ask me to extend, or over-extend, myself for another, and I can perform at a consistent 110%. Ask me to spend time taking care of myself, and, as good as that sounds, it just as much confounds. How would I take time for myself when others still have so many needs, when there are more school or work assignments that call my name? Even if I did decide I need time for myself—that this would help me in overcoming my eating issues—words like self-compassion and self-care sound nice, but I couldn't begin to really wrap my head around what that actually looks like in my life. I'm certainly not able to think about self-care in my daily life!"

Kat speaks for many of us. For many of us who struggle with food, our struggles have roots in learning to put others first, to be giving and sweet and nice, and to always put people at ease. Those can be lovely lessons that help us support others and get along well in the world.

Yet these lovely lessons have a darker underbelly. They teach us that we are capable and we are good when we give to others. This can eventually undermine our sense of self and our trust in our capabilities. I mean, if we want to know and trust ourselves, we need to put the focus, support and help on ourselves. To the extent that isn't okay to do, we learn to keep the focus of our activities on others.

Meanwhile, we subtly learn to distrust our deepest instincts and wisdom. It's important that this is subtle, because otherwise we could, we would, rise up against such treatment. Instead, we come up with an ingenious solution to such a conundrum.

We learn to play big for others and play small for ourselves. We learn how to never be "full" of our convictions, passions, proclivities—our essence. Instead, we end up turning to food to fill us up in ways it cannot do, so that no matter what we eat, we are never full. Because food can fuel our lives, but it can't fulfill our lives.

Another way we learn to play big for others and play small for ourselves is to seek to control people, places, and situations. If we can restrict the variables, we can feel safe in a potentially unsafe world. We end up restricting food in our efforts to regulate our world—finally finding at least one thing that we can perfectly control, our eating. Yet too little food will be better at making us light-headed than it will be at making the world a safer place. So we continue to control our food, and wait and hope for the day when the world is finally safe, so we can present our true selves. But that day never comes in this scenario because our true selves need the freedom and space to move beyond restriction, to let go of control, in order for that unique individual essence that is you to play big.

So here is the good news about all of that. We only have to pay attention to our plates and the seven practices to change this state of affairs. Food, once your biggest stumbling block, and your "only real problem" becomes your active personal assistant. Your journey with eating, your struggles with eating, lead you to the path where you can choose to play big in the ways that are most deeply true for each of you.

This is a terrifying, electrifying, wondrous proposition. That behind what is sweet and nice and always wants others to feel comfortable, behind your search for control and acts of rebellion, is a true self that is always patiently waiting for you to come home. A true self that is waiting to show you your beauty, your essence, and the pathway to your truly unique contribution.

As Kat began to incorporate the seven practices for healthy eating into her life, she suddenly began taking an hour for a massage instead of a fifteen-minute stress fix at the McDonald's drive through. She replaced gobbling the afternoon chocolate bar at her computer with a ten-minute walk outdoors and deep breathing. Slowly, yet surely, this elusive thing called self-care began to happen for her. As she took better care of herself, she found energy and excitement in taking care of her family and her work. Slowly, yet surely, she found a sense of freedom from emotional eating.

Now is the time to invest deeply in your freedom! Let's go!

"There is a vitality, a life force, an energy, a quickening, that is translated through you into action, and because there is only one of you in all time, this expression is unique."

—Martha Graham

The Seven Practices
for Lifelong
Healthy Eating

4

Sixteen-year-old Rebecca stands in the kitchen holding her iPhone in her right hand. She is staring intently at a cupboard. She takes a step towards it and then stops. She lifts the phone and re-reads a text message from her best friend. It's the message in which her best friend says, "Oh hey just wanted to let you know that Jimmy asked me out. You don't mind that I go right." Rebecca scowls at the phone. Her friend knows she has liked Jimmy since junior high. She can feel the heat in her face, and looks in the mirror for just long enough to see that her face is really red. She doesn't say to herself that she's angry, yet her face glows redder as her anger rises.

A period at the end of that sentence! Her best friend did not even ask this as a question. Even though the whole situation, as far as Rebecca is concerned, is completely out of the question.

Suddenly, she dashes the remaining distance between her and the cupboard, flings it open, reaches inside, and grabs a Twinkie. She holds it in her hand and looks doubtful. Then, a feeling of serenity comes over her. She anticipates the sweet taste that will make everything else go away. She walks down to the family room and turns on the television. Just as she is about to open the Twinkie and enjoy its creamy sugary goodness, her mother enters the room and checks out the situation. "Oh, honey," her mother says. "You don't really want to eat that do you? I mean, you've been doing so well on your diet."

Rebecca, a sweet, mild tempered kid, looks at her mother. Her face goes dark. She takes the Twinkie and throws it across the room. It hits the wall. When the impact hasn't changed the shape of the Twinkie, Rebecca picks it up and smashes it between her hands. She opens the door to the backyard and throws the flattened Twinkie into the yard.

"Honey", her mother says. "Is something wrong?" To this question, Rebecca's answer is a scream. Rebecca runs out of the family room and into her bedroom slamming the door behind her. She flings her body onto her bed, sobbing into and beating upon her pillow with unadulterated frustration.

Now, I'm not saying that your proclivity for comfort food is based in an anger you haven't noticed, nor a resentment you've never thought—or thought very briefly, and then had to dismiss. Maybe you've pounded a pillow with unadulterated frustration.

Maybe you're sucking it up in the way that conforming to expectations means sucking up the food so you can keep living in line with expectations.

A simple truth is: We knew how to eat as babies; this was natural. So when our eating behaviors fall out of sync with healthy living, we need to reconnect to what we already know. As babies, we were whole and imperfectly perfect. We stumbled around, giggling at our failures and our successes. We barely knew how to tell them apart. This attitude is again what we need when we learn to eat well.

But how?

Great question.

This is where the seven practices for lifelong healthy eating come into our discussion. The next section of the book will give details of each practice. Here is an overview:

Practice One: The Foundational Triangle. The first practice is learning to use The Hunger Scale, The Connection Scale, and choosing an Accountability Pal. The practice of using these tools grounds your journey in quick-to-accomplish check-ins as you practice awareness of your mind, body, and spirit. This will help you understand your eating patterns and make the process of what to eat and when clear and simple.

Practice Two: Slow Eating. The second practice is learning a method for slowing the process of eating your food. This practice will help you enjoy your food (there are no good or bad foods), eat healthy portion sizes, and truly savor each bite.

Practice Three: I Have a Choice. The third practice helps build awareness of the moments before eating where you can consciously choose what is best for you to eat. This practice will help you feel more freedom in your eating life and behaviors.

Practice Four: The Art of the Pause. The fourth practice is learning several methods for taking a pause when you are feeling stressed and want to turn to emotional eating to mitigate your stress. This practice will help you put all of the other practices into use and save you a bunch of heartache.

Practice Five: Practice Not Perfection. The fifth practice is creating a mindset wherein you deal with the pesky perfectionist. You will learn how to develop an attitude of practicing toward your eating goals each day, and (Hang on to your hats!) walking yourself through the moments where you are failing or less than stellar with kindness and grace. This practice will help you be kind to yourself when you are eating in a balanced way, and will help you keep going if you fall out of balance with your eating.

Practice Six: Building Intentional Relationships. The sixth practice is learning to look at food as a relationship. This practice helps you take an up close and personal look at food as a friend. Is food acting as a good, positive friend or a lousy one who often leaves you feeling crummy after you've spent time together? This practice will help you become very intentional about your food friends and your people friends as well.

Practice Seven: Your Guardian Grace Advisor. The seventh practice is learning how to access your own inner wisdom based on "hearing" the voice of those who have helped to guide you. This practice will help you know that you've got this and you're never really alone.

Are you ready to break free from emotional eating? Let's get to it!

Practice One: The Foundational Triangle

I *'ve been running at top speed all day, and I'm starving!* Sarah thinks to herself. She opens the refrigerator and briefly contemplates making a salad. The distance to the vegetable crisper drawer suddenly lengthens. The idea of preparing food for herself in addition to food for her husband and the kids becomes overwhelming. "It's mac and cheese for all of us!" she decides. She grabs the cheese from the fridge, opens the cupboard and takes out pasta and a bag of potato chips and begins munching on the chips and cheese as she cooks.

By the time dinner is ready, she's on the eating treadmill. She's not sure if she's hungry, but there's food so she eats it. After the family is fed, her husband does the nighttime routine with the kids as she hops onto her computer to get a few work emails answered. It's late and she's tired and doesn't really want to be back in front of the computer, so she grabs a package of cookies to make the task more pleasurable. An hour later, she reaches into the package and is surprised when it is empty. *Enough,* she thinks, and she decides to do something about how she is eating.

Like Sarah, maybe you've reached the point where you're ready to figure out emotional eating. Great! Congratulations! You've decided to do it—to dive into figuring out stress eating, emotional eating, mindless mind-numbing eating, under-eating, overeating, binge eating, angry eating, rebel eating.

This is where we will begin by learning three simple tools which will become the foundation of freedom and relief from non-healthy eating. You will use these tools to practice quick check-ins with yourself so that you become aware of your physical hunger and your emotional state before you begin to eat.

I'm going to be straight with you. When I say simple tools, I mean simple. But I do not necessarily mean easy. The task may not be easy, but it will be worth it as you begin to experience when, why, and what you're eating.

Using these tools takes only minutes, five to ten at most. These may become some of the most tedious moments of your life. And also some of the most enlightening. You will use these tools to look for patterns in your thoughts, feelings, sense of

confidence, and sense of connection in the current moment—
the moment right before eating.

You might be thinking, *What? Every time I eat I have to think about these things? What a drag!* But then again, there is that relief and freedom thing that sounds pretty delicious. So, without further ado, let's meet our first practice.

The first practice is learning to use three tools: The Hunger Scale, The Connection Scale, and your Accountability Pal. Using these practices diligently will help you connect to your roots before you lift your fork. An eater who is rooted and connected to her life is a different eater than one who is frantic or unaware or stuffing or restricting food.

The Hunger Scale

To use the Hunger Scale, simply rate your actual physical hunger from 0—10. Zero means pretty much starving. Ten means pretty much stuffed. To develop patterns of healthy eating, try to stay within 3—7 on the hunger scale. If you dip below a three, then you will tend to overeat because you have a sense of deprivation.

A study took young men in their early twenties who were healthy, trim, and had no eating issues. They put them on a calorie restriction diet for six months. After that time, these men overate for the next five years, and did develop weight problems. A crummy study, I get that! The important point for the purpose of practicing the hunger scale is to avoid getting below a three rating, as that is likely to trigger a physiological reaction of wanting to eat too much and too fast. When we pay attention to not going below a three rating on the hunger scale, it will help us to prevent overdoing it later.

If we plow on after we've reached a seven, we are eating beyond what our bodies need and truly desire for nourishment. Many people, upon using the hunger scale, notice immediately how often they eat beyond a seven. They will try to break down the space between six and seven into very small fractions. "I think I'm at a 6.8, so I can still keep eating." Notice your resistance or disappointment at getting near a seven.

I've found that as we practice checking in with the hunger scale, people make it their own in two ways. First, they may tweak the numbers. A previously bulimic eater likes to stop at her six, because she feels that getting to a seven triggers an overeating response. Second, as eaters practice the hunger scale, they begin to find that the urge to eat outside of the three to seven range begins to slip away. We begin to reclaim a relationship with ourselves in which eating is about nourishment and enjoyment of our food. To help that become a reality, we need to access our second fundamental practice: The Connection Scale.

The Connection Scale

The Connection Scale puts you in touch with your thoughts and feelings as they are before you pick up your fork. It consists of two fill in the blank questions and five "I feel" questions that are quickly rated between 0 and 10.

The questions are:

1. My most prominent thought that I'm thinking/ thinking about now is _____.
2. My most prominent emotion that I'm feeling now is _____.

The feeling scale, with zero at low intensity and ten at high, is:

I feel connected to joy. 0 = Joy? Seriously? Life sucks, dudette. 10 = Hell, yah! Life is good!

I feel connected to others in ways that are fun and supportive. 0 = I need a woman cave big enough for one. 10 = That was fun! I'd like to do it again.

I feel connected to my goals. 0 = Goals, schmoals! 10 = I've got this!

I feel connected to school and/or work in ways that are fulfilling (not exhausting). 0 = I'm a stress mess! 10 = This is challenging, but so worthwhile!

I feel confident (that things will work out, in my abilities, in my relationships, that I can handle the next task in front of me). 0 = Deer in headlights paralysis. 10 = I feel pretty, and witty, and wise!

For each of the "I feel" ratings above, the zero and ten ratings and the prompts in number five are guides. It's important to follow your intuition about your rating, not overthink it! If there is a thought worthy of follow up, by all means give that thought attention and journal time. But when using the scale before eating, make it quick.

Keep a record of your answers. You will use this to look for patterns.

At the end of the meal, you will also record if you successfully stayed within the three to seven hunger scale rating and you will note if you need to access the third fundamental practice: Your Accountability Pal.

Your Accountability Pal

Your Accountability Pal is someone you will choose to help support you on your journey to enjoy heathy eating. You'll identify a person you want to call when tempted to engage in old behaviors. Then, you will call them! Not text, PM, email, or send smoke signals. You'll pick up your phone and use it to connect your voice to the voice of another person. (Even if you get connected to their voice on voicemail.)

Here are steps and things to consider when choosing your Accountability Pal:

Step One:
- Choose one or more people. Reach out to ask them to be your Accountability Pal.
- Choose a person/people who are
- Trustworthy
- Straightforward
- Supportive
- Available

Step Two
- Describe where you are now and where you want to go.

This doesn't have to be a fantastic goal; it can be "I want to quit bingeing at night." Ask your Accountability Pal if they would be willing to provide support for times when you're feeling scared or slipping into old patterns. Ask them if they are willing to learn the language of the Hunger Scale and the Connection Scale. Your Accountability Pal doesn't have to be a trained professional nor have similar goals to you. It will be someone with whom you can share vulnerable moments, and who knows you well enough to do verbal hand-holding when you need it.

We've learned our first practice. Perhaps you feel a tremor of exhilaration, a twinge of fear, a wall of doubt, a ray of hope. When you begin to deal head on with something that has dogged you for too long, and honestly seek solutions that have evaded you for too long, something has already shifted toward the positive. Now, you just practice.

"Whatever you can do or dream you can, begin it. Boldness has genius, power, and magic in it."
— **Johann Wolfgang von Goethe**.

Practice Two:
Slow Eating

6

Linda is eating a donut as she heads out the door for a day full of to-dos. She runs errands for five hours, then stops by the Taco Time drive-through on her way to visit a friend. She has a music rehearsal in the evening, so she eats a power bar for dinner on her drive. After rehearsal, she's feeling hungry and pulls a quick u-turn on the way home to pick up a chocolate milkshake at McDonald's. The milkshake leaves her with a vague feeling that she hasn't actually eaten, so when she gets home she makes a sandwich and eats it while she checks social media before bed.

The fact that she has not once sat down with her food without multitasking doesn't dawn on her. She's a busy gal, with a full life, and paying attention to her food is not a part of her daily routine. But it is a big part of why she struggles with food portions, food choices, and a yo-yo pattern of weight gain.

Slow your roll, baby. Slow. Your. Roll.

Whether you're about to eat an actual roll or anything else, your next practice is that of Slow Eating. I'll give you a step-by-step description, so that you can easily perform this practice. Here's the part where I may be glad that you're a book away from me—that is that you're reading this book and we're not together—because the moments of your first few slow eating practices may not be your finest.

Go ahead, direct all of that resistance and thoughts of how ridiculous this is right at me. I'm a book away, and I can take it. I will also be there when you discover that less is more, that less food that is more specific to what you really want and need to eat, is far more satisfying than mere quantity.

Except, not at all, at first. Because, well, the restrictions, or the wild abandonment of them. Nevertheless, this is the next practice, so Brave One, let's get going.

You're getting ready to eat. You've checked in with your Hunger Scale rating and Connection Scale ratings. It must be time to dive in to your meal, right? Not quite yet, Wise Grasshopper.

Next, we practice Slow Eating. This will not be your forever eating experience, yet in the beginning of behavior change, it's important to practice this to the best of your ability.

Slow Eating redefines the steps to beginning to eat. You will need a dose of patience, a remembering that you really want a change in your eating, and a journal of your choosing to record thoughts while in-between bites.

Here are the steps:

- **Step One:** Be here, now. Eat only at the table, not in the car or on the fly. Don't nibble before nor pick at what might be left on your plate after you eat.

- Feel your feet on the floor. Feel your body in the chair. Get comfortable. If you want an A+, imagine that your feet connect you to a deep tree-like root structure that is stable and secure, and extends deep, deep, deep to the center of the earth.

- **Step Two:** Take three deep breaths. Inhale deeply, filling up your lungs, and exhale slowly and fully.

- **Step Three:** Smell your food. That's right. Smell what's on your plate. Register if it smells good, not so good, actually bad, has no discernable smell to you.

- **Step Four:** Take a bite. One bite. Set a timer for one minute. During that minute, reflect on your experience of the food. Is it satisfying? What textures and tastes do you notice? Is what you're experiencing what you expected? Hang tight until the timer goes off before your next bite. Take notes of your thoughts—any thoughts, don't judge them—and record them in your journal. (If you're doing this in a group, there can be a specific person who keeps the timing, so that the timer is not as jolting. If you're alone, please set a nice tone to your timer to make the sound as pleasant and non-jolting as possible.)

- **Step Five:** Repeat step four. After every two bites, check in with your Hunger Scale Rating. When you get to seven, stop eating. (Not after seven bites, yet at the 7 of your Hunger Scale. A little bit of hilarity and panic when these got confused.)
- **Step Six:** Clear your plate, without further nibbling.
- **Step Seven:** Check in: Do you need to contact your Accountability Pal? If so, do it. Now. If not, turn your attention to something other than eating. Preferably something enjoyable.

One thing I've particularly enjoyed is what clients have said about the practice of slow eating. After a meal together at a retreat, Janet said, "I couldn't believe that I didn't enjoy eating bread. I mean, me and bread go back a long way. But when I slowed down, it didn't taste that great. That was unbelievable to me. And what was even more unbelievable is that the vegetables on my plate tasted better." Next, Carole spoke up, "I thought that I overate to get energy when I'm overworked and stressed out. But when I do Slow Eating, I see how eating makes me more tired if I'm already overextended." That remark prompted Julie to share, "I learned I didn't want to just eat anything and everything, I wanted to eat things that tasted delicious to me." Natalie had looked a little sad as she listened, and decided to share this with the group, "I learned that overeating is a kind of violence to my body and also that I use overeating to punish myself. I couldn't figure out why I'd be punishing myself, but it made me sad. Slow Eating helped me see what I was doing and let me feel those feelings."

There was a pause, the group listening and every person nodding. After a moment, Valerie spoke up, "When I started Slow Eating, I became aware that I love a little food, a lot." A bit of laughter and more nodding. Roger, brave man in a group of women, was the last to speak, "I didn't think I could do it. I was convinced I couldn't do Slow Eating. No way. No how. Now, I think, is there any other way to eat? I don't think so!"

We've learned the Slow Eating practice. Perhaps you feel skeptical that this endeavor is becoming a little bit larger or stranger or different from what you expected. Maybe your old ways weren't so bad after all? I've never been so convinced that my struggles with restrictive eating and bulimia were not really as big a deal as I was making them as the moment I had my hand wrapped around the doorknob of my first therapist visit. "You're overreacting. You're making too much out of this. You don't really need to be here. It's not too late to leave, and just not show up for the appointment. It's not like you even know this therapist, so just bail." Those were the thoughts in my head, and no thoughts in my entire life had ever been more believable. I still don't know how or why I turned the doorknob and stepped into her office. At some level, I must have been in touch with my pain and discomfort, but that isn't what I was thinking about then. I was thinking all of the thoughts above, along with the very scary thought of "don't name it, for goodness sakes, don't talk about this out loud."

So do your best to turn your doorknob, and let a little of the light and hope for change come in. Take lots of deep breathes, and be here, now. And remember, now you just practice. The seven practices will help you get to healthy and balanced eating. There is nothing to get right or perfect. There is only practicing as best you can.

As you practice, you learn about portion distortion. A lovely client recently was successful in her goal to get on top of healthy eating habits. "I learned my biggest enemy is portion distortion," she said confidently.

Her remark triggered the scientist in me. I grabbed my experiment notebook, put on my safety goggles, and got to work. First, I filled a cup that I inherited from my grandmother with water. Then I poured the water into a measuring cup. Four ounces. Next, I filled a cup that I use for my morning coffee. Then I poured the water into a measuring cup. Twelve ounces.

In the course of two generations, portions have grown three sizes! And so have a lot of people. Apparently, it's not the dryer to be blamed when our jeans are a wee bit tight! This is good news—to realize that portion distortion is a part of our struggles with food. When four ounces meant one serving, we were satisfied, and happily lived within that norm. When twelve ounces becomes the norm, we begin to feel cheated if we're eating less.

Recognizing that you have "supersized" your food intake norms, you can begin to correct the portion distortion in your life, which often includes re-portioning your work load and number of commitments as well. When you re-normalize to a reasonable portion of food, you can turn your energy to supersizing your heart and goals, so that growing your heart and goals three sizes bigger becomes your new normal.

"If you want to fly, you have to give up the things that weigh you down."

– Toni Morrison

Practice Three:
I Have a Choice

I mentioned earlier there are no good or bad foods, and before I get going on this chapter I want to address the question that is most likely on your mind. If I'm saying there are no good or bad foods, then what is to stop you to going to comfort food when the going gets tough. Geez Louise, don't I realize that's exactly what you're trying to stop doing?

I do realize that. But here's the deal: Going to what you call comfort food can be okay if you are conscious about what you're eating and how much of it is going into your body. The point, which can be a bit counter-intuitive when you are dealing with what you've identified as comfort food, is to get out of black and white thinking that is the culprit behind up and down weight cycles, and obsessive thinking about food. It is a thinking that limits your experience of food choice and expression of choice in your foods, and will sabotage your efforts.

That said, you are completely free to decide certain identified comfort foods are off the table, both literally and figuratively, for you. This expands your sense of choice rather than limits it.

When you engage your sense of choice, you begin to unravel the drama around food and simply see it for what it is. Here is an apple. Here is a cookie. The apple doesn't stand for good, truth, and all that is honorable. The cookie will not kill you. These last two sentences are actual quotes from a client describing how she felt about those foods before she began to practice Choice. That was the thinking at which she had arrived. Now, let's take a look at how you may have arrived at the thinking about good and bad foods.

If you struggle with food, there is a very high likelihood that you will have been introduced to the idea that there are good and bad foods. You might have learned this as a child by watching your mother diet and choose salad while salivating over the pasta on everyone else's plate. You might have learned this from going on low-calorie, restrictive diets. You might have learned this way of thinking from feedback in your environment that insinuates that your weight isn't okay. You may have learned this kind of thinking from the subtle and not so subtle looks that pronounce judgement in the form of a suggestion that you might wanna' switch out carrot sticks for corn chips. However you got there, you arrived at the place where you view some foods as good, and others as bad: veggies are good, pizza is bad; fruit is good, cake is bad.

We make the assumption that certain foods are better than others. And in that moment, we become a slave to stressful thoughts about eating and choice. When our choices are defined for us, limited by others and then by our own internalized limits, we rebel or toe the line. Our rebellions become homages to restrictive eating or they lead us to become out of control eaters. When we toe the line, we develop resentment and also begin to second-guess ourselves. We want pizza not vegetables, so we begin to gnaw away at our capability to trust that we can solve the simplest of troubles: what to eat. If I can't know with great certainty that I can be trusted to properly feed my own body, how can I become a confident and fulfilled woman?

Bringing back your ability to choose is the next practice.

Years of research tells us this kind of black or white thinking, which includes thinking that there are good or bad foods, is detrimental to healthy eating. This thinking hurts and leads to losing and gaining, and often regaining more weight. Many of us enter the yo-yo weight cycle, which keeps us in alternating states of exhilaration, despair, and dress size.

The first and foremost tenet of the practice of Choice is that there are no good or bad foods. No foods are off limits. Yet, you do need to be savvy and concerned with the overall nutritional content of your food choices.

You, Brave One, on this mission to change your eating behaviors, have full choice of what you eat. For some, the unlimited exploration of what you can eat is like a joyful puppy bounding about a newfound meadow. It is exhilarating and wonderful and free!

For others, this unrestricted idea causes anxiety. In these cases, you will need to draw your own parameters around what to eat, order, put in your cupboards. For a few years, Ben and Jerry's Super Fudge Chunk Ice Cream could not enter my home. Nor Fritos. I was beginning to feel a freedom around food, yet certain things, certain specific foods while not bad, were not allowed because they could throw me into a state of white-knuckling it or encourage a binge that I'd later regret.

During the time I kept them out, I kept experiencing more joy in less food. In every bite. It was weird that my eating, which had defeated me so often, was helping me to find a way to set limits for myself and experience satisfaction.

As you do the practice of Choice, you'll choose whatever you want to eat. You'll notice if what you expected to experience meets your expectations.

Here you'll notice whether the food meets your expectations and hopes and desires. You'll notice if you're meeting your own expectations and hopes and desires. Just notice.

You choose, then notice the outcome of your choices. You choose, then notice the thoughts and feelings surrounding your choices. In *Hamlet*, William Shakespeare writes "There is nothing either good nor bad, but thinking makes it so."

Because, Brave One, you are wise and wonderful and capable of making strong positive choices for yourself. You are infinitely more than you think. Yet what you think matters because from your thoughts, come your choices. As you embark on the fundamental practice of Choice, you become picky and specific about all of your choices, from what's on your plate to what's on your mind. There are no good or bad foods, no good or bad thoughts. Some foods, and some thoughts, are just better at getting you where you want to go.

"You are infinitely more than you think. Yet what you think matters."

– Robin Rae Morris

Practice Four:
The Art of the Pause

I've been talking about emotional eating, the theory that when we eat when we're not physically hungry, we are "eating our emotions." No one who has ever struggled with eating needs a theory to tell her that. Newsflash: Your feelings of boredom, confusion, anger, sadness, disappointment—I could go on, but I'm guessing you get the idea—those feelings may be behind your food struggles. Gee, I never thought of that said no troubled eater ever.

What do I do about it? Now that's an entirely different question, which leads us to the next practice: The Art of the Pause. Sometimes a pause is only a micromoment long. Yet, every pause is an opportunity. Actually, every pause is three opportunities: to give yourself time to rethink what you're about to do in the next moment, to break a habit or pattern that impedes your life or your goals, and to handle life without turning to food to mitigate your stress.

For the purpose of learning to pause, and to appreciate the pause, you're going to explore the nature of emotions as they relate to learning to pause. The English word emotion is derived from the French word *émouvoir*, which comes from the Latin word *emovere*. In Latin, the e means energy, and movere means motion. Let's break that down for modern times.

Our first step is to add a slash inbetween e and motion. E is all about energy. Our various emotional states create energy, and the greater the emotional experience, the greater the amount of energy we will feel surging through our bodies. Motion, on the other hand, has to do with movement and action. In this case, motion is how we express the energy that arises from our feelings.

When emotional energy becomes the undercurrent pulling you toward out of balance eating, the best thing you can learn to do is pause. A pause puts moments, sometimes mircomoments, between the energy of your emotions and the action that follows. Too often we take action just seconds after feeling an intense emotion. Here, we mistakenly believe that our energy must be expressed as soon as possible. Here are two examples:

Your ideas are overlooked by your boss in a meeting, and so you immediately start inhaling from the bowl of M&M's a co-worker brought to the meeting.

You put on an outfit you love, and when your partner gives you a questionable look, you grab a piece of cold pizza from the fridge.

Often we need only the slightest of pauses to stop the unhealthy eating cycle before it begins. The pause gives us time to consider all possible options before taking action. Hitting the emotional pause button can be summed up in the following formula:

E (emotional energy) {PAUSE!} Motion (expression)

Now that the formula is clearly presented, we need to discover the Art part of our fundamental practice of The Art of the Pause. The Art lies in how to take a pause when your emotions are pulling you downstream on a rapidly moving raft. Here are five pause techniques that have been wildly successful for those who are working toward healthy eating habits. Take a test drive and see which ones work best for you.

1. **The Lifesaver Tool (Created by W. Doyle Gentry, PhD)**

   When you are experiencing a strong emotion, suck on a Lifesaver and wait until it dissolves (no chewing!) before taking any action. This will take Type-A folks about four minutes and the rest of the population about six minutes. While that sounds like a short amount of time, what you are likely to do four or six minutes after your initial emotional response is drastically different than what you are likely to do immediately after feeling strong emotions.

To understand why this tool is so helpful, consider that the sucking response is one of the first actions we perform as babies; we quickly learn to associate it with comfort and sustenance. Also, while a Lifesaver doesn't have a lot of calories, it does have a pleasant, sweet taste. Experiencing this range of associations—sweetness and comfort—right when you're also feeling a surge of anger or sadness, for instance, is confusing for your human brain and forces you to pause. When you're wound up, buying a little time for your brain is priceless.

2. **The Sniff Tool (Created by J. LaPointe, PhD in life)**

Go outside and take a sniff. Actually, take three of them—breaths, that is. Let your body take the lead in helping you relax. Most intensified emotional states produce contractions in the body and constriction of the blood vessels. Deep breathing does the opposite by helping your body relax and your blood vessels expand. Since your mind and body is are interconnected, you'll find your mindset also relaxes and opens to new possibilities.

3. **The I-Need-a-Moment Tool**

When you are experiencing a strong emotion and it is driving you to gobble up any and everything in sight, recognize it as a red flag. This is not the time to eat your hurt, anger, or frustration. Nor is it the right time to act impulsively, even though it will feel like the perfect time to hit the drive-through or the pizza place.

The red flag is screaming, "Eat! EAT! EEEEEAT!" When you feel this way, say, "This is a red flag that I need a moment before I do anything, especially before I start eating." When you're focused on solving issues right away using food as the solution, you will forget it is perfectly appropriate, and often necessary, to take a moment. Give yourself a moment, thereby creating distance between you and the situation, and you and a foot-long submarine sandwich. Return to the situation when you're able to deal with it with a calmer, more level-headed approach.

4. **The Do-Anything-Else Tool**

When you're at your wit's end, overcome with emotion, and ready to lash out, you can create a pause by doing anything other than what you're about to do. Stand on your head, sing a song, recite a poem, or take a walk. And keep standing on your head, singing that song, reciting that poem, or taking that walk until you feel confident you can choose to take an action that will have a positive outcome. This isn't rocket science, but it's definitely challenging. Not only will this technique help you stay out of trouble, but it will also allow you the chance to pause and love yourself. Give yourself permission to be less than perfect. Give yourself space. Give yourself grace.

5. **The Play-Dead Tool**

A client once asked me, "What do I do if none of the other pause tools work for me?"

I answered, "Play dead."

The client looked stunned, but I said, "Don't knock it till you've tried it."

We humans go through extreme emotional experiences. Maybe you feel bored, provoked, tired, sad, lonely, and angry all at once, or maybe there are a host of other emotions that are hitting you on a grand scale. When this happens, I think of a comic strip that shows two couples at a dinner party. The hosts are so hopelessly bored yet stuck that they lie down in the middle of their living room and play dead. The other couple slowly notices and makes the decision to leave. When push comes to shove, when you don't know what to do, when you only know you don't want to exacerbate a bad situation or return to old patterns, just play dead. Hit the floor. It may not be the most elegant solution, but it will save you heartache.

It's important to know that The Art of the Pause will become one that protects and honors your choices around food. As you continue to practice, you will make a surprise bonus discovery: From pausing before eating comes the feeling you are a pause-worthy person. Pause. And your true presence appears.

"Practice not-doing, and everything will fall into place."
– Tao Te Ching

Practice Five:
Practice, Not
Perfection

Lindsey, a former collegiate gymnast and current client, is a lovely young woman who is comfortable looking at me and lying to my face. During our conversation, I say, trying to maintain a casual, off-handed, non-alarmist tone, "You do realize that human beings are not capable of being practically perfect in every way, every day, all day long."

"Yes, I do realize that," she replied. Aha! Liar, liar, pants on fire!

I slowly lower my glasses to the tip of my nose, and peer over the top of the frame at her.

Because she's a nice kid, she cracks. "Okay, I realize that other people don't have to be perfect. But I have to. I mean, it's what I'm supposed to do! I've spent twenty-three of my twenty-six years on this planet trying to get a perfect ten score. I don't know how to just stop demanding perfection from myself. It's just not okay with me to fall below the perfect ten, even though I do of course."

"And then what happens?" I ask, glasses back in the right place on my face.

"I start eating food that makes me feel better or I deny myself food until I've done something perfect enough to deserve it." She sounds angry as she begins to talk, yet begins to softly cry when she gets to the words "deserve it."

I ask her if she'd like a hug and she nods yes. I want to wrap my arms around her and protect her from the part of her that is her worst eating enemy. The part that will not allow her peace from the struggle of perfection. The part that will not allow trying her best and doing her best to be good enough, ever. The part that invariably brings her right back into the thick of her struggle with food. "Your best is good enough, and you are enough." I say to her in almost a whisper. These are delicate moments, and I know that the tables have turned a bit because now she's pretty sure that I'm the one who is lying. Within a year, Lindsey came to believe that her best was good enough, and once even said her not best was the best she had to give that day.

Once she began to be enough, to be imperfect and okay with that, the hold that food had over her days slowly, yet surely, slipped away.

Many who struggle with unbalanced and emotional eating also struggle with perfectionist tendencies. Not everyone expresses it as clearly and staunchly as Lindsey did in her session. Yet clients often express a subtle terror about making a mistake that only comfort food, or the denial of it, can shake.

Then there is the double whammy of feeling bad about being less than perfect and falling back into old behavior patterns, finding yourself behaving strangely and unhealthily around food. Again.

These are the moments in which you will be tempted to give in to despair and self-loathing. These are the moments in which you will want to convince yourself that you will never achieve a healthy relationship with food. That other people may be successful at this, but you must have been in the ladies' room when that particular skill of healthy eating abilities was handed out. These are the moments in which you will want to, once and for all, accept defeat and let yourself finally just give up, and go up another clothing size or three.

Yet, Brave One, you haven't come this far to fall into a dark ugly pit of disliking yourself nor doing the disservice to yourself of giving up on beautiful you. You have arrived at the point in which you need to embrace Practice, Not Perfection. This starts with an acknowledgement of what choices you've made that didn't turn out well, and moves directly, swiftly, and immediately into a place of self-forgiveness.

I remember mentioning this to a client who had been stuck in a week of binge eating after several months of healthy eating. I gently reminded her of Practice, Not Perfection. I gently reminded her about the self-forgiveness part.

"Forgiveness? Is that like talking nice to myself about being a complete loser?" When I confirmed that talking nice to herself was indeed part of it, she replied firmly, "Well, if I were to simply talk nice to myself when I failed again at this food thing, it would be a short trip to the place where everything in my life would go to h*** in a handbasket." Oh, the things we will believe. Oh, how we will put up with the hellish bad treatment of ourselves around our eating issues. Oh, how that very bad treatment can keep us locked into the patterns we're trying to change.

The harsh reality is that when we are being unkind to ourselves by bingeing or restricting food, we become unkind to ourselves in other ways. When it comes to something as fundamental to our very survival as food as literal nourishment, we find that the way we treat ourselves about food becomes the way we treat ourselves about life. Eating too much food often comes with over-doing it with commitments. Restricting food intake in regimented ways can lead to being stiff and inflexible in day-to-day situations. Instead of knowing how to bend with the winds of life, we more often break. Or at least, feel broken and defeated. This is all the more reason to become skilled at Practice, Not Perfection.

I realize that it is often easier said than done. Again, yet another reason to become skilled at this practice. If you, like this client, find it difficult to talk nicely to yourself after you've failed to hit eating perfection, I have a challenge for you. Try it. The talking nice to yourself part, that is. Next time you fail to choose healthy eating, or perceive that you have failed at making balanced food choices in any way at all—in a giant, fantabulous, kind of epic fail or in a small, only I know but I'm disappointed with myself integrity fail, be nice to yourself.

Let's take a non-food related example for just a moment, because sometimes our harsh attitudes about our eating issues make it more difficult to apply this practice to ourselves. Let's take an example of a young child learning to ride a bicycle. The kid inevitably falls off the bicycle at some point. The parent walks over to the child. The parent does not say, "You idiot. You can't do this right. You can't really do anything right! Other kids half your age are better at this than you are. That's it, no more bicycle for you!" The parent does not say that, yet many of us from the ripe old age of about twelve begin to talk to ourselves in this manner when we perform below perfection. And the deal with that self-talk? Well, it turns out that your self is listening.

Inside of those who struggle with balance in eating is what I call the inner eating-critic. This is that voice that thinks it is helping you to become a healthy eater by using the following three methods: nagging you constantly about your real or perceived failures, keeping up the negative play-by-play of your behaviors, and comparing you to others or to a better version of yourself, as in not the version you are being in this moment.

Let's throw the inner eating-critic a bone, shall we? After all, it thinks that if it keeps up this methodology, you'll eventually get a magical reward of being good enough at eating correctly. There is a fly in the ointment of the inner eating-critic's plan: nagging, negativity, and comparison will not produce a sustainable positive result.

Plus the inner-eating-critic forgot someone important. It forgot the inner eating-kiddo in you who is sad, lonely, frustrated, scared or all of the above. Remember our kiddo who just fell off the bicycle in the above example? What the parent actually says to her sounds more like this: "Are you hurt? Did you get scared? Everybody, and I mean everybody, who learns to ride a bicycle falls off when they are learning. You'll get this. How about we shake off the fall and try it again."

Your deepest self, the part below your relentlessly harsh inner eating-critic, that part of you that is heart and intuition and that loves you and all that you are, is hearing all of the judgements and criticisms you're bringing upon yourself.

After years of coaching, and sitting with clients, I don't believe that your deepest self believes these things, yet I do believe it is saddened by hearing them. That deepest self remains your biggest fan, contains your essence, and unconditionally loves you. But it will run for cover, hide under a rock, do whatever it needs to do to protect its survival, if it needs to protect itself from your busy, judging, disapproving inner eating-critic.

The conscious mind soaks up the negative self-talk of your inner eating-critic like a ShamWow soaks up a bad spill. All of the judgements, all of the criticisms, all of the failures become reasons you don't deserve love and kindness. They become the backbone for why you must push yourself to overeat, overwork, over-rebel in a frantic effort to get back to your essence.

It's nice to know that your essence is always there, patiently waiting for you to return, patiently waiting to lighten your load. In this way, your essence is a little like the parent in the bicycle example. In that example, there was an inquiry of are you scared? Are you hurt? Are you okay? This was followed by reassurance, and the invitation to try again. This is Practice, Not Perfection. And don't worry, if you try this and everything goes to h*** in handbasket, I promise you that your inner eating-critic has more than enough experience not talking nicely to yourself after a perceived fail, that you will retain the skills to do it. But my hope for you is that once you give Practice, Not Perfection a bicycle spin around the neighborhood of your life, you'll choose to support, reassure, and invite yourself to give balanced eating one more try.

> *"No matter how you feel, get up, dress up, show up, and never give up."*
>
> **– Lori Sanders**

Practice Six:
Intentional
Relationships

10

Rebecca is bummed. On the outside she seems fine, but inside, within her most intimate relationship—the one she has with herself and eating—she is miserable. "It used to be that other people—friends, family, coworkers, a random person in the mall—made me nervous," she explains. "I had a talking doll when I was a kid, and when you pulled the string, she would say phrases like 'I have butterflies in my tummy' and 'I'm just afraid of everything!' And that's exactly how I felt! Maybe that's why I loved that doll so much ..."

"Shrinking Violet!" I exclaim. "I loved her too! Although looking back, she was so nervous and sad; she had zero self-confidence."

Rebecca laughs. "Yeah, she was a hot mess! Nothing like the smug, self-satisfied, 'I'm amazing!' dolls that my children have today. I used to think that doll was the only one who really understood me," she says almost wistfully. "But now all those relationship issues are gone. I like spending time with my friends, family, husband, and even the people at my work. It's the internal stuff that's all messed up now, it's really my eating that is the most messed up."

She elaborates, "I can't eat right. I've tried diets, but they only made me more miserable. With the dieting I'd get skinny, but then as soon as I stopped dieting, I'd get way fatter! What a joke. Another joke –on me! Oh, and get this: I just finished my master's degree in nutrition! With honors! I'm a living comedy hour."

"Gaining weight, and now you have a degree that's bogus." I slowly consider this aloud before adding perkily, "Well, at least you haven't lost your sense of humor."

Suddenly Rebecca isn't laughing anymore. In fact, she looks mad. "Excuse me? Are you even listening?"

"I am listening," I say. "But enough about me; let's get down to your relationships."

"Okay, really? I knew you didn't get it!" Rebecca is growing angrier.

Before she becomes completely exasperated, I get serious: "Humor me a minute. What if we looked at your messiness and struggles with food as a relationship?"

I remind Rebecca that she used to be an emotional see-saw around her friends, family, and coworkers: bouncing between false confidence, extreme insecurity, and angry rebellion. Her relationships were unbalanced and exhausting at best and resulted in dramatic misunderstandings at worst. I remind her that she successfully found ways of creating boundaries and enjoying her relationships.

"Okay, I get what you mean," Rebecca nods. "This does feel similar. I don't have those people problems anymore, but I still feel that way about food. One minute everything's okay, but the next it's terrible! I become like an overly critical parent, demeaning myself in the hopes that criticism will help me make smart choices. Then when that backfires, I rebel and eat out of control. If I were to compare it to a relationship, it would be like having good sex with the wrong guy. It's all fun in the moment, but afterward you feel scummy. And obviously he doesn't really care about you."

Out of aggravation comes a plea for moderation with the way we see and use and relate to food. Out of frustration comes a desire for freedom.

Rebecca is on to something important, so I continue. "The kind of relationship you establish with food will have consequences, which we learn about through trial and error. For instance, if you eat way too much, you might find yourself losing self-esteem and a lot of money on a new wardrobe. But there's no reason to beat yourself up; in fact, that usually keeps you from learning, since you're too busy searching for a big enough stick with which to club yourself."

I can see Rebecca is connecting with my theory, so I keep going. "Instead of slandering yourself, try examining the results of your choices and letting those guide your future decision making in order to bring about the consequences you desire. For instance, our grandmothers and science both say that a balanced diet—one with a variety of foods eaten in moderation—is the best way to achieve a healthy body, increase energy, and expand creativity. As a master nutritionist, you know that scientific research—and your grandmothers—have found that diets don't work. In fact, people almost always regain more weight than they lose. And they lose heart as well when they realize that being thin doesn't magically lead to happiness and that they denied themselves for no reason."

"Oh, yeah!" remembers Rebecca. "Nothing like being thin and unhappy to send ya' to the store for chocolate."

"Don't forget the frozen pizza," I add.

"Do I look like someone who's ever forgotten the frozen pizza?" she asks rhetorically. She has put on sixty pounds in the past eighteen months.

I pause and consider—and then reconsider—asking her if she wants to talk about her weight gain. Instead, I propose, "Why don't we think of different foods as friends? They have the potential to be a supportive friend or not. When you're hanging out and having a good time, it's easy get swept up in the moment and think, this friend is awesome. I love hanging out with her. We should do this all the time!

"But try to remember how you feel after hanging out with her. If you still feel good, wonderful! But if you don't, then it's time to think about ways you can spend time together that don't end up making you feel bad. If you can't, then it's time to say goodbye to that friend.

"Our issues with food help us work on our boundaries so that we can stay present in the presence of any person or thing without breaking down or compromising ourselves—without feeling 'icky' afterwards. Too much food leaves us with a hangover. But there's no such thing as trusting ourselves too much. It's joyous to wake up feeling good about ourselves, our integrity intact, knowing we have made healthy choices."

"I seriously get it," Rebecca says.

"Good," I reply. "To stay in integrity, it helps to understand the difference between intention and impulse. Let's compare and contrast, shall we?"

Intention	Impulse
Sense of clarity, clear choices and direction	Sense of urgency
Sense that things will be okay; a gentle confidence about the present and the future	Freaking out because you fear your needs won't be met
Feeling relaxed	"Gotta' have it now!"
Filled with joy, peace, and purpose	Scurrying around; filled with anxiety, nervousness, and a sense of doom
Feeling balanced and whole	Feeling out of balance; going to extremes

Two weeks later an energetic Rebecca shows up for our appointment. "Treating food like a relationship has helped me see when I act out of intention or impulsivity. Acting impulsively feels like it helps in the moment, but it really creates a great big 'ick' afterwards. Deciding to act with intention makes me feel good about myself, the way a good friend does. And, I don't want to make any big proclamations here, but thinking of food as a relationship might be helping me to be a better friend to myself."

Like Rebecca, many of us who are emotional eaters discover (or re-discover) what it feels like to be a kind and wonderful friend to ourselves as we practice healthy eating. Through practicing healthy eating, and becoming friends with yourself once again, an interesting thing will happen. Once you are your own best eating friend, you will tend to pull in better quality support and friends.

Your ability to see food as a relationship becomes a way of seeing how to choose the best relationships to help you grow. Those are the relationships that make you laugh and also make you want to show up as the powerful woman you were always meant to be.

"When you are your own best friend, you don't endlessly seek out relationships, friendships, and validation from the wrong sources because you realize that the only approval and validation you need is your own."
– Mandy Hale

Practice Seven:
Your Guardian Grace
Advisor (GGA)

11

We have arrived at the last of your seven Fundamental Practices. This is where you call in help. You have your Accountability Pal(s), yet this wise and graceful presence is a little different. This is one you can access and turn to any time. This Guardian Grace Advisor is there when we think to ourselves, "This craving is intolerable." She is there when you feel, "I can't stand it! I'm too powerless and lost in dealing with this situation."

Sounds good to have 24/7 access to such a person, right? Here's how. Imagine you're working at central casting for a huge movie studio. You have access to historical figures, wizards, fairy godmothers, friends, mountains, lakes, rivers, talking animals, and more.

Next, invite your senses to bring the Guardian Grace Advisor you need now to light. Feel the Guide's strength, patience, love, unconditional acceptance. Identify the qualities you need in this moment that your guide possesses. Then, write the name of your GGA at the top of a page of your journal or a document file. After that, write your question to your GGA. If you have more than one question, ask them one at a time. Write out the response in a Question and Answer format.

I'll share an example from one of my journals.

GGA: Deborah

           Qualities she brings: Warm smile, trusts in me, helps when I'm stuck, helps access my wisdom, fills in wisdom when I don't get it, grounded presence, believes in living our faith in daily life.

Q: I'm afraid that even though I feel strong now, the strong pull and impulsive nature of when I feel that a craving is intolerable will throw me off course with healthy eating. How do I handle these situations?

GGA: So during your success and enlightened moments, you're planning for failure and despair?

Me: Maybe I'm just a good planner....

GGA: Or struggling to be in the moment.

Me:	There is that. I could enjoy this wonderful moment, and not worry so much about the moment that isn't here yet.
GGA:	There you go.
Me:	(hesitating)
GGA:	Let's talk about your question a little more.
Me:	Thanks.
GGA:	You're worried about being in the throes of craving. That you won't know what to do.
Me:	Exactly.
GGA:	(Laughing) Didn't you write a chapter about The Art of the Pause?
Me:	Maybe…
GGA:	Use it, the practice.
Me:	What if it doesn't work for me? What if it only works for others?
GGA:	Now you're talking about a whole different question.
Me:	True.
GGA:	Let's stay with the first question. What's the last example of practicing the Art of the Pause?
Me:	Play dead.
GGA:	Remember the comic?
Me:	Yes. (Now I'm grinning and not so worried).

GGA:	You can do that.
Me:	That wasn't a question, was it?
GGA:	No.
Me:	It can be delightful to struggle. I mean, in that growth happens in the struggle.
GGA:	And in enjoying the moment. All moments.
Me:	Thank you!

I remember feeling so much lighter, so free of worry after this "conversation." I also remember that I wrote it during a workshop, and my first thoughts about doing this exercise were "I suck at these kinds of exercises and I don't even believe they work."

Turns out neither of those thoughts mattered. What mattered was that I gave it a shot, gave it a try. What mattered was that six minutes and ten seconds of writing changed my mood from fear to hope. Six minutes and ten seconds, hardly enough time to order an Uber delivered pizza, let alone go through the motions of overeating, then being stuck with guilt and shame, and the original fear. And this was an exercise I didn't believe in. Imagine when we actually start believing in our ability to hold tight, instead of bolt into the well-known world of food obsession and compulsive eating.

When we hold tight, and try, each of us can access the wisdom of our Guardian Grace Advisor. Be ready for them to show up in various forms. Know that when you call, when you ask your most pertinent question, they will answer you with insight, humor, a directive, or a hunch.

We are meant to heal, to grow, to flourish and thrive, to love. These seven fundamental practices will set you on your way. While we each have a path to walk, remember you don't have to go it alone. There is grace and support built into your journey—you need only to ask for it to appear.

"You're never so lost, that your Guardian Angels can't find you."

– client and workshop participant

Put Down
the Chocolate
Covered Peanuts

At one food retreat, I finally spilled the beans. Or more specifically, I talked about the chocolate covered peanuts, Let me tell you about that in a bit more detail. When I was coming out of the thick of eating out of balance, I would still purchase two pounds of chocolate covered peanuts to take with me when I needed or wanted to purchase new clothing. I hadn't quite got to the part where I trusted my decisions, so food was still a companion. Sometimes I ate the chocolate covered peanuts while I shopped. Sometimes I just held onto them, an extra weight in my purse, knowing I could munch, munch, munch if it was getting progressively difficult to find jeans that fit.

What I didn't take into account is that every person in modern society has problems finding jeans that fit. (I'm going to let that sentence be its own paragraph.).

For me, and most who have struggled with eating, there is a lesson in holding onto the chocolate covered peanuts. That yes, if you eat your way through purchasing new clothes, then you're likely to have to buy newer new clothes that fit your expanding, chocolate covered peanut indecision.

This makes it important to review the seven practices for lifelong healthy eating and realize that these things that are occurring with a high degree of importance and drama are just that: drama raised to an infinitely larger reaction that includes food as a solution.

Some of the obstacles that occur include:

- Falling into old behavior patterns, even when you wake up each morning feeling determined to eat in a healthy way

- Struggling to do the Seven Fundamental Practices on a consistent basis

- Feeling lost when you try to sort out emotions, feelings, and troubling experiences after you've decided you won't "eat them away."

- Having a relapse (binge, restriction, or other) after a period of healthy eating and emotional freedom

- Ending up at the fast food drive-through or grocery store when you absolutely were not, absolutely not, going to stop there

You are capable of changing your eating behaviors, developing new ones, and becoming your true self on your own. It's just that it's so much harder to do any of those things alone.

There is strength in numbers, even in one plus one, when we seek change.

When Carol came to me she was struggling with emotional eating because she had no support. She had gained and lost forty pounds three times. She joined my twelve-month program and found the accountability, support, and new friendships she needed to maintain her weight loss when facing obstacles.

Carol's journey is a good reminder that when you face obstacles on your own it's likely that the bag of chocolate covered peanuts is going to come out again when you hit a roadblock. Make sure to see where you can find the support you need to maintain healthy eating and keep growing your life.

The Unexpected Epicurean

13

Louise is a twenty-year award-winning restrictive dieter and binge eater extraordinaire. She has taken down her gold medals and been free of these behaviors for five years.

In those five years, she left her job as a senior project manager and opened a restaurant. Wait, what? Wouldn't those career choices have gone the other way around?

One would think. Our rational minds say the last place a person who has suffered with their relationship with food should end up is in a kitchen. Then again, that's what we get for thinking primarily with our rational minds. Don't get me wrong, our rational minds are amazing and capable of incredible feats. Yet, sometimes they just don't get it. (Remember the therapist who suggested I binge on fruit in chapter one?).

As Louise practiced each of the seven steps, she became very picky and very curious about what she was eating. Once, she had eaten to numb emotions, rarely thinking too much of the taste, texture, experience of her food. If it was good, that was great. If it wasn't too good it was there for her. An outstanding pizza and an average tasting pizza were still pizza after all.

But all that began to change. The average tasting pizza wasn't worth her bites on the Hunger Scale. Average or below average tasting food slowly but surely just couldn't cut it.

One day, in a moment of saying no to store-bought chocolate cake offered at a work meeting, Louise had a revelation. She had become a picky eater! She, who once was more than happy to eat to be eating, was saying no to chocolate cake.

And, simultaneously in that moment, she became curious about what food she was now willing to say yes to. She realized she wasn't as clear on the answer as she thought she might be. She could address categories—cheese, bread, fruit, vegetables, baked goods, and yes, chocolate and pizza. But the specifics eluded her.

Confident in her use of the Hunger Scale, the Connection Scale, and all of the practices, she began to explore the world of cheeses, baked goods, and bread making. She began to seek out locally sourced vegetables and fruits. And the world of food became fascinating!

A previous attitude of "I just love cheese!" became "I just love aged Gouda paired with a perfectly ripened Anjou pear." The more she explored, the more specific she became about food, and the more she truly loved food. And you know that when you truly love something you treasure it, not overwhelm it with endless, or restrictive, quantities. You treasure the quality of the thing you love.

If we are restricting our access to food, or cramming our faces with half a chocolate cake before we realize we're in the act of eating, are we really loving food? If we loved food wouldn't we be slowing down and savoring time with the thing we say we love?

When you love someone, you pay attention. When you love someone, you have an incredible, enduring, fantastic curiosity about them. You yearn to truly understand their mind, heart and spirit. Sounds lofty, yet I'm talking about the everyday ways a person moves, talks, walks, decides, hurts, and laughs. What grabs their interest? What are their fears, their beliefs, and their passions? When you love someone, you understand their sadness, or grumpiness. You celebrate their successes. When you love food, you pay attention to the taste of it, you notice if the allure meets your expectation, you notice if something tastes better, or worse, than you expected.

When you love someone, you spend time. You spend time but don't feel exhausted by it. You spend time as to notice each moment, appreciate each moment. You spend time in a way that brings out an infinite number of possibilities for sharing love, light and laughter in a single moment. This harkens back to slow eating. When you love food, you slow down and spend time with it. Your food isn't an afterthought that you cram inbetween other to-do items on your list. Your food becomes worthy of your time, and in return, time with your food becomes time well spent.

When you love someone, you listen. I'm talking about a particular kind of listening, where listening is aimed at understanding the heart of another. It's listening with fresh ears, even if you feel like you've heard it a million times before. It's the kind of listening that waits to digest what you've heard before you respond so that you can respond, and not react. How? By being curious, asking questions, and making sure you understood what the other person wanted to communicate. And so with food, you listen. You listen to your experience of eating. When is it stressful? When is it stress free? When do you want to eat when you're not physically hungry; what is your heart, mind, and spirit saying to you? When you listen to the desire to eat, what do you hear?

When you love someone, you protect them and enjoy them. Protecting those you love takes a lot of care. You want to let them fly free, yet not so free as to fall. You have learned seven practices. They are practices because they protect you from old eating habits, from going to one extreme then another to restrict or over-eat. You have learned you can simply love food and choose enough, and not too much, of it.

I think of a former client, Linda. She was very regimented in her eating but would blow out of her restricted patterns in a big way. How big? Her weight yo-yoed up and down to the tune of seventy-five pounds. She would say her problem was that she just loved food too much.

Yet when I proposed the idea of loving something based on Paying Attention, Spending Time, Listening, Protecting, and Enjoying One Another, she realized that by that criteria, she'd given up loving food long ago. As she made the seven practices a daily effort, she began to get clarity on really loving food.

She began to spend time with her food and to pay attention to it. That led to her wanting to listen and enjoy time with being in her perfectly imperfect body. Linda had a renewed sense of sensuality about food, and this translated into a renewed sense of sensuality about her body. This made a big difference in her romantic life, which had been stalled out when she was stuck not liking her food choices nor her body.

Linda's story reminds us that once we begin to really love food, we naturally begin to love ourselves and the people in our lives more fully as well.

After incorporating these seven practices into your life, you can have the same outcome as Louise and Linda. You can start to say yes to those foods that fuel you and no to those that leave you feeling depleted. You can start to heal your relationship with food and see it as something to care for.

14

Permission Slips:
Saying No, Saying Yes.

Your journey with food is also a journey about life. I'm fond of the statement, "Travel is how you get from one moment to the next." It is in each moment that you do the Seven Fundamental Practices. It is in each moment that you give yourself permission to experience choice, to pause, to create intentional relationships, to call upon help.

Once upon a time, each elementary school child needed a permission slip to miss class or go on an exciting field trip. Now, you are able to create a new kind of permission slip—one that says it's okay to grow into your unique self and play big in the world. Each moment you can write a permission slip that allows you to say "No, I can't come to class today," or "Yes, I can go on an exciting adventure today."

In each moment, you can give yourself permission to say No. To say no to the foods, people, things, places, and thoughts that no longer serve you. In each moment, you have the possibility to quit apologizing for the past. You have arrived in a present moment where you can choose to give your permission to say no.

Along with that comes the permission to say yes. Yes to the right food at the right time. Yes to less work, yes to more rest, yes to more joy, yes to a crazy idea, yes to a trip you've longed to take, yes to connection, yes to the moment.

In the moments when you speak your truthful no, and heartfelt yes, you experience freedom and relief. Yet, Brave Ones, you didn't come this far to do this only for yourself, though that is a wonderful, and wise, starting point. As you give yourself permission to be free from emotional eating, you will give others around you permission to be free to face their problems as well. You may never speak a word, yet your presence will change your environment, because you've done the tough work of changing inside, one no and one yes, at a time.

I wish for you all the joy and success and permission you'll ever need. And if you need a little support to keep going, you can find it at www.robinmorriscounseling.com. It sometimes takes a village, and there you'll find your tribe waiting to support you.

Acknowledgments

To the Morgan James Publishing team: Special thanks to David Hancock, CEO & Founder for believing in me and my message. To my Author Relations Manager, Margo Toulouse, thanks for making the process seamless and easy. Many more thanks to everyone else, but especially Jim Howard, Bethany Marshall, and Nickcole Watkins.

About the Author

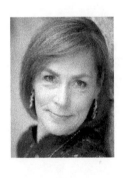

Robin is a licensed mental health counselor who enjoys private practice in Woodinville, Washington. She loves the beauty of the Pacific Northwest, biking, hiking, snow skiing and traveling. She has worked in community agencies, private and public schools, and has been a dance teacher and theatre director for kids five to ninety-five.

In all of her work, Robin is most concerned with the transformational process for each individual, and providing opportunities for deep connections between individuals. Her varied professional career gives her a unique, creative and easy to relate to style. She encourages clients to become self-empowered and to access their innate creativity.

Robin has a Masters Degree in Existential Phenomenological Therapeutic Psychology from Seattle University, in Seattle, Washington. Don't be afraid of that last sentence, it just means that her therapeutic training focuses on the importance of being present and showing up to live our lives fully.

To learn about counseling, consulting and speaking opportunities, please visit

Website:RobinMorrisCounseling.com
Email: Robin@RobinMorrisCounseling.com
Facebook: https://www.facebook.com/RobinRaeMorris/